Proven Natural Ways to Lower

High Blood Pressure

30 Proven Natural Superfoods To Control & Lower Your High Blood Pressure

By *Louise Jiannes*

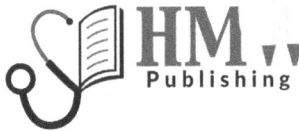

HM ᵥᵥ
Publishing

For more great books visit:

HMWPublishing.com

Download another book for Free

I want to thank you for purchasing this book and offer you another book (just as long and valuable as this book), "Health & Fitness Mistakes You Don't Know You're Making", completely free.

Visit the link below to signup and receive it:

www.hmwpublishing.com/gift

In this book, I will break down the most common health & fitness mistakes, you are probably committing right now, and I will reveal how you can easily get in the best shape of your life!

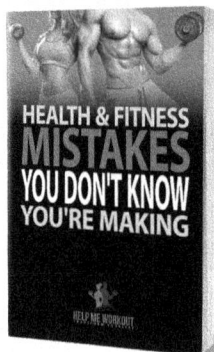

In addition to this valuable gift, you will also have an opportunity to get our new books for free, enter giveaways, and receive other valuable emails from me. Again, visit the link to sign up:

www.hmwpublishing.com/gift

TABLE OF CONTENT

Introduction   **12**

Chapter 1 – Overview on High Blood

Pressure   **16**

How Can High Blood Pressure Occur?   17

Chapter 2: The Dangers of Having High

Blood Pressure   **20**

Damage to your Arteries   21

- Damaged and Narrowed Arteries   22

- Aneurysm   22

Damage to the Heart   23

- Coronary Artery Disease   23

- Enlarged Left Heart   24

- Heart Failure   24

Damage to the Brain   25

- Transient Ischemic Attack (TIA)   25

- Stroke   25

- Dementia   26

- Mild Cognitive Impairment   27

Damage to your kidneys   28

- Kidney Failure   28

- Kidney Scarring   29

- Kidney Artery Aneurysm   29

Chapter 3: Causes and Symptoms   30

Essential Hypertension   31

Secondary Hypertension   33

Chapter 4: Preventive Measures for High

Blood Pressures   35

Preventive Factors You Can Control   35

- Maintain a Normal and Healthy Weight   36

- Eat a Balanced Diet   37

- Cut Back Sodium Consumption   37

- Limit Alcohol Intake   38

Have a Regular Exercise   38

- Monitor Your Blood Pressure   39

- Changing your Bad Habits   39

Chapter 5: Proven Ways to Control High Blood Pressure Without Medication   **40**

What about if you already have that sickness in you?   41

How Can One Benefit From the Natural Treatment?   43

- Weight Loss   44

- Improved Stamina and Energy   44

- Reviving Youthfulness   45

- Controlling Hypertension   45

- No Side Effects!!!   46

Natural Ways to Control High Blood Pressure

Without Medication   46

- Step #1 – Walk, walk, walk!   47

- Step #2 – Inhale, Exhale!   48

- Step #3 – Take More Potassium, Reduce

  Sodium in Your Diet   48

- Step #4 – Add Cocoa to Your Diet   50

- Step #5 – Alcoholic Beverage Helps, Too! 51

- Step #6 – Avoid Caffeine   52

- Step #7 – Avoid Working Too Much!   53

More Alternative Treatments to Include in

Your Diet!   54

- Selenium   54

- Beta-Glucan   55

- L'Argine   55

- Fish Oil or Flaxseed   56

Chapter 6: Herb Remedies: How Can They Help to Normalize Your Blood Pressure   **57**

Herbal Remedies for High Blood Pressure

                                      57

- Arjuna (Terminalia Arjuna)   57
- Dandelion (Taraxacum Officinale)   59
- Cayenne (Capsicum Annum)   59
- Ginger (Zingiber officinale)   60
- Guggul (Commiphora Wightii)   61
- Garlic (Allium Sativum)   61
- Reishi (Ganoderma lucid)   62
- Hawthorn (Crataegus app)   63
- Hawthorn (Crataegus Laevigata)   63
- Celery (Apium Graveolens)   64
- Cocoa (Theobroma Cacao)   64

- Valerian (Valeriana Officinalis) 65

- Broccoli (Brassica Oleracea var. Italica) and Dark Leafy Greens 65

- Turmeric (Lucuma Longa) 66

- Gingko Biloba 66

- Olive Leaf Extract 66

- Jaundice Berry 67

- Cayenne 67

- Red Clover 67

- Alfalfa 68

- Parsley 68

- Gooseberry 69

- Onion and Honey 69

- Fenugreek Seed (Trigonella Foenum-Graecum) 69

  - Lowers Blood Cholesterol 70

- Reduces Risks of Heart Disease   70

- Keeps You in Shape   71

Chapter 7: Stress Management:

Empowering Mind and Body   **72**

The Connection Between Stress and Long-term

High Blood Pressure   72

Activities that Can Reduce Blood Pressure   75

Make Your Schedule Simple   75

Be Conscious of Your Breathing   76

Do Regular Work Out   77

Meditate   78

Develop Good Sleeping Habits   79

Be Optimistic   81

Chapter 8: How Meditation Can Help in

Lowering High Blood Pressure   **83**

Managing your Health, Saving Your Life!   87

A Way To Do Your Meditation Exercise   88

Conclusion   **93**

INTRODUCTION

The rising number of people affected by high blood pressure had brought awareness to the public but being aware of the sickness or its presence is not enough to exclude you from its deadly fang.

For decades, this sickness had been ignored and overlooked because of its silent symptoms which earned it the title of being the "Silent Killer" but as government's efforts are driven towards minimizing if not eliminating its presence; attention to this illness is being brought forward to the public.

If you are one of the many people, who are not comfortable living with the idea that you could be affected by this illness without actually knowing it. This book, "*Proven Natural Ways to Lower High Blood Pressure*" will equip you with the knowledge of high blood pressure and how to reverse it naturally without the use of medications.

Furthermore, while we are discussing the treatment of high blood pressure, we should also be aware of its preventive measures. Know all the essential facts about this silent killer to live a healthier life!

Also, before you get started, I recommend you **joining our email newsletter** to receive updates on any upcoming new book releases or promotions. You can sign-up for free, and as a bonus, you will receive a free gift. Our *"Health & Fitness Mistakes You Don't Know You're Making"* book! This book has been written to demystify, expose the top do's and don'ts and to finally equip you with the information you need to get in the best shape of your life. Due to the overwhelming amount of mis-information and lies told by magazines and self-proclaimed "gurus", it's becoming harder and harder to get reliable information to get in shape. As opposed to having to go through dozens of biased, unreliable and un-trustworthy sources to get your health & fitness information. Everything you need to help you has been broken down in this book for you to easily follow and to immediately get results to achieve your desired fitness goals in the shortest amount of time.

Once again, to join our free email newsletter and to receive a free copy of this valuable book, please visit the link and signup now:

www.hmwpublishing.com/gift

CHAPTER 1 – OVERVIEW ON HIGH BLOOD PRESSURE

High blood pressure is one of the primary contributing causes of death in the United States. According to the recent report released by the Center for Disease and Control Prevention, about 75 million American adults have high blood pressure. To give you a quick calculation, that's one out of every three adult Americans or around 29% of the American population. Approximately $46 billion is spent by the nation each year to cover health care services and medications. This also includes missed days of work due to hypertension.

Symptoms of high blood pressure are sometimes so mild that it's hard to detect. However, its results can be deadly and therefore must be taken with the utmost concern. Untreated, high blood pressure, also known as "hypertension can damage and can leave scars to the arteries which can also be found even in people who are normally calm and relaxed. The "Silent Killer," as it carries no initial symptoms, is a long-term illness, which can eventually lead to complications and death.

HOW CAN HIGH BLOOD PRESSURE OCCUR?

High blood pressure is the impact of the blood created against the wall of the arteries as it circulates inside the human body. The blood pressure is determined by the amount of blood pumped by the heart against its resistance as it flows through the arteries.

When there are some blockades like cholesterol build up, scarring or plaque in the arteries, it affects the elasticity of the arterial walls and narrows the way of the bloodstream, thereby creating more pressure as the heart pumps harder to get the blood through so that it can reach the different parts of the body. Such increase in pressure can damage the muscles and valves of the heart and may result in heart failure. Damages to the vessels supplying blood and oxygen to kidneys and brain eventually create a negative impact on these body organs.

Too much pressure in the blood vessels and arterial walls can cause serious problems. Healthy arteries are usually semi-flexible tissues and muscles that are fine, smooth, elastic and stretchable, so blood flows smoothly through them when the heart starts to pump mildly. However, when there are blockades, the heart is forced to pump more thereby stretching the walls of the arteries, and if done too much, it could break the lining of the arterial walling. Once blood vessels are broken, it could lead to stroke, kidneys malfunction, peripheral vascular failure or heart attack, which causes death to the majority of its victims.

It is, therefore, essential to keep your blood pressure at a level to reduce the risk of blood vessels from getting overstretch beyond its limit. Uncontrolled blood pressure increases the risk of more serious health or medical problems to occur.

CHAPTER 2: THE DANGERS OF HAVING HIGH BLOOD PRESSURE

High blood pressure is steadily increasing in modern societies due to an unhealthy lifestyle. This can be very disturbing if you are not fully aware of its implications in your health condition, but if you do, you can look for useful options to reverse its effects.

High blood pressure can silently do some serious damage to your body system long before the onset of symptoms. Taking it for granted can result to a disability, a life of suffering, and even a severe heart attack. People who are left untreated of high blood pressure die of ischemic heart disease or reduced blood flow. Others die of stroke. A shift in lifestyle and treatment can help control your high blood pressure to reduce these life-threatening risks. Now, let's take a look to some of the damages it can cause to your body.

DAMAGE TO YOUR ARTERIES

When your arteries are healthy, they are flexible, elastic, and strong with a smooth inner lining along the walls to let the blood flow freely as it circulates the body. This is a vital process as it supplies nutrients and oxygen to vital tissues and organs. When the bloodstream is clogged, it causes an increase in pressure in the arterial wall as the heart pumps vigorously to let the blood flow in. As a result, you could be experiencing the following:

- *DAMAGED AND NARROWED ARTERIES*

  When you have an unhealthy lifestyle, your body can collect fats from your diet and store them in your arteries, clogging the flow of the bloodstream and your artery walls become less elastic. This limits the flow of blood in your body.

- *ANEURYSM*

  Eventually, the constant pressure of blood against the weakened artery lining may cause a part of the wall to form a bulge. This condition is called "an aneurysm." An aneurysm can rupture anytime and can cause internal bleeding in any of your arteries, but mostly it occurs in the aorta or the largest artery in your body.

DAMAGE TO THE HEART

Since your heart pumps blood to your body, uncontrolled high blood pressure can do damage to your heart in many ways.

- *CORONARY ARTERY DISEASE*

  This condition affects the arteries that supply blood to the body. The disease narrows down the arteries and limits the blood to flow freely through the arteries. When you have this illness, you can experience irregular heart rhythms known as (arrhythmias), chest pains or an irregular heart attack.

- *ENLARGED LEFT HEART*

  When your heart is forced to exert vigorously to pump blood into your body, it causes the left ventricle to become stiffen or thickens (left ventricular hypertrophy). These changes also limit the ventricle's ability to pump blood thereby increasing the risk of a heart failure, heart, attack and sudden cardiac death.

- *HEART FAILURE*

  Eventually, the strain on your heart caused by the high blood pressure weakens your heart muscles and makes them work less efficiently. If this continues to go on, this condition will just wear out your heart. Your heart will wear out in time and fail and if there's some damage caused by heart attack, they add more to the existing problem.

DAMAGE TO THE BRAIN

Like your heart, the brain depends on the supply of blood to nourish it so it can work properly to survive. However, when there is high blood pressure, it can cause problems including what we have here below.

- *TRANSIENT ISCHEMIC ATTACK (TIA)*

   Considered as a "mini-stroke," this condition is a temporary disruption of the blood supply to your brain. Transient Ischemic Condition is often caused by atherosclerosis or a blood clot. Both of these can arise when there is high blood pressure, and the presence of the TIA is a warning that you're at risk for a full-blown stroke.

- *STROKE*

   When part of your brain is deprived of oxygen and nutrients supplied by your blood vessels, it will cause the death of your brain cells. So, when you have high blood pressure that is left uncontrolled or neglected, this can cause the narrowing, rupture or leaks in your blood vessels leading to the brain. High blood pressure can likewise cause blood clotting in the arteries blocking the blood flow to your brain and causing a stroke.

- *DEMENTIA*

  This condition is associated with problems in cognitive abilities – thinking, speaking, reasoning, memory, vision, and movements. There are various causes of dementia including vascular dementia, which is attained through narrowing and blockage of the arteries that supply blood to the brain. It can also result in a stroke that causes an interruption in the blood flow leading to the brain. In any of these cases, it's the high blood pressure that mainly causes it.

- *MILD COGNITIVE IMPAIRMENT*

  There is a transition stage, which occurs between the changes in understanding, and memory as one grows old and the more severe problems develop when one gets, for example, an Alzheimer's disease. Like dementia, this results from blocked blood flow when high blood pressure damages arteries.

DAMAGE TO YOUR KIDNEYS

Typically, it's the function of your kidneys to filter excess waste and fluids from your blood, though this process depends on your healthy blood vessels. When high blood pressure injures your blood vessels leading to your kidneys, it may cause numerous types of kidney diseases (nephropathy). If you have diabetes, this can even worsen the damage.

- *KIDNEY FAILURE*

  Kidney failure is caused by high blood pressure as it brings damage both to the large arteries leading to your kidneys and the tiny blood vessels (glomeruli) within the kidneys. Damage to either of these two affects the normal function of your kidneys hindering it from efficiently filtering waste from the blood. In the end, a dangerous level of waste and fluids can accumulate in your body and may ultimately require dialysis or a kidney transplant.

- *KIDNEY SCARRING*

  Glomerulosclerosis is a type of kidney damage caused by scarring of the glomeruli (glue-MER-u-li). The glomeruli are tiny clusters of blood vessels within your kidneys that filter fluid and waste from your blood. Glomerulosclerosis can leave your kidneys unable to filter waste efficiently, leading to kidney failure.

- *KIDNEY ARTERY ANEURYSM*

  This is a type of an aneurysm leading to the kidney. One potential cause of this disease is atherosclerosis, which damages and weakens the artery wall. In the long run, a weakened artery can cause a section to form an aneurysm, which can rupture anytime and cause a life threatening internal bleeding.

CHAPTER 3: CAUSES AND SYMPTOMS

It's not easy to identify the exact cause of high blood pressure, but numerous factors and conditions that may somehow have contributed to its development.

Here are some among them:

- Obesity or overweight

- Lack of physical activity

- Too much consumption of salt and alcohol

- Smoking

- Genes and family history including high blood pressure

- Unmanageable stress

- Chronic kidney ailments

- Thyroid and adrenal disorders

- Sleep apnea

ESSENTIAL HYPERTENSION

In the United States, more than 95% of reported high blood pressure cases, the underlying cause is not determined. For this type of high blood pressure, people in the medical world call it as the "essential hypertension."

Mysterious as it is, essential hypertension has been linked to specific risk factors. High blood pressure tends to affect more males than their female counterparts and is likewise observed to run in the family.

Moreover, age and race also play a vital role. African Americans living in the United States are twice as more likely to have high blood pressure compared to Caucasians, but the gap decreases at around age 44. Many black women have the highest reported incidence of high blood pressure at the age of 65 and above.

Other factors that affect essential hypertension are diet and lifestyle. The link between salt and high blood pressure has long been established. Japanese people living in the northern islands of Japan are known to consume more salt per capita than people in the rest of the world, and they've got the highest incidence of essential hypertension. Conversationally, who don't use salt to their food have no traces of essential hypertension.

People with high blood pressure are hypersensitive, in other words, this means that even a small excess of salt added to what is typically needed by the body can send their blood pressure to soar up. Other factors that count in the presence of essential high blood pressure are an insufficiency in calcium, magnesium, and potassium, chronic alcohol consumption, obesity, and diabetes.

SECONDARY HYPERTENSION

Contrary to essential high blood pressure is the Secondary High Blood Pressure or "secondary hypertension." This type of high blood pressure, the direct cause is somehow pinpointed, and kidney disease ranks the highest among the many causes of secondary hypertension.

This type of high blood pressure can be triggered by tumors and other abnormalities, which cause the adrenal glands to produce excess amounts of hormones that elevate the blood pressure.

The factors that can send blood pressure to rise include:

- Pregnancy

- Birth control pills particularly those that contain estrogen

- Drugs that constrict blood vessels

CHAPTER 4: PREVENTIVE MEASURES FOR HIGH BLOOD PRESSURES

Making an extra effort to prevent the onset of high blood pressure can help in the reduction of stroke, heart attack, and many other serious illnesses that can lead to death. If you are at risk for high blood pressure, it's best for you to take these preventive measures.

PREVENTIVE FACTORS YOU CAN CONTROL

Some factors like, age and genes including family medical histories are elements that are beyond your control. Therefore, if you want to prevent the onset of high blood pressure, you need to focus on the risk factors that you can change. We are not able to do something about our age or what constitutes our

DNA, but we can always change our lifestyle for a better and healthy one.

Here are some ways to consider in shifting to a healthy lifestyle.

* *MAINTAIN A NORMAL AND HEALTHY WEIGHT*

    Maintaining a healthy weight is crucial when it comes to hypertension. Overweight and obesity can lead to more complications, which can eventually lead to death. People who are overweight need to lose weight and if you are of average weight, then avoid adding more pounds. Finally, if you are carrying extra weight, lose as much as ten pounds to help prevent the occurrence of high blood pressure. There are online resources to help you know your ideal weight and your body mass index (BMI).

- *EAT A BALANCED DIET*

  Eating a healthy balanced diet can help keep your blood pressure under control. Eat foods that are rich in potassium while keeping a limit on calories, fat, sodium, and sugar. DASH Diet is known to help in managing high blood pressure.

- *CUT BACK SODIUM CONSUMPTION*

  The higher the sodium intake you have, the higher the blood pressure rises. Therefore, it is better to cut down on your sodium intake by avoiding foods that are high in sodium content like packaged foods and processed food. It may also help to prevent adding salt to your meals.

- *LIMIT ALCOHOL INTAKE*

  Drinking too much alcohol thickens the blood and therefore creates more pressure for the heart to have it flowed smoothly and freely. Thus, avoid having more than a drink in a day.

HAVE A REGULAR EXERCISE

It takes activity to make one healthy, and physical activity is crucial when referring to high blood pressure. The more exercise you have, the better. However, even a little bit of exercise can do so much to lessen the risk of hypertension. Start doing a moderate amount of exercise for about 30 minutes. Starting by training two to three times a week is an ideal target to begin.

- *MONITOR YOUR BLOOD PRESSURE*

    After you have done with the ways stated above, make sure that you regularly monitor your blood pressure. To do this, you can either go to a clinic or do this at home. Since hypertension often shows no apparent symptoms, only the blood pressure reading can give you a definite measurement of your blood pressure. Blood pressure reading in the range of 120-139/80-89 millimeters of mercury (mmHg) puts you at an increased risk of developing high blood pressure.

- *CHANGING YOUR BAD HABITS*

    Finally, take a look at your lifestyle and see what among your habits needs to change. Try conquering small goals like eating fruits and vegetables instead of junk foods in between meals. Make these habits as part of your daily routine.

Chapter 5: Proven Ways to Control High Blood Pressure Without Medication

Although we have introduced some preventive measures to get away from having high blood pressure, still we know it is not that easy to make a 360 degrees shift in your lifestyle. With the kind of modern life we have today, when almost everyone is always on the go, we fill in our stomachs with ready-to-eat foods right out of the package. We know that these foods are far from being healthy and unless you are determined to change your ways, you need to refrain from eating theses kind of foods.

WHAT ABOUT IF YOU ALREADY HAVE THAT SICKNESS IN YOU?

As I have stated, high blood pressure is a sickness that must not be ignored. Deaths related to high blood pressure run to almost 100,000 each year and is still rapidly increasing. Some people just ignore their problem while others choose medications with harmful effects. But, nowadays, the majority of people resort back to the use of simple natural remedies to treat high blood pressure. There are many natural remedies proven over the years to combat high blood pressure.

Before considering drug medication for your hypertension problem, take note of the following facts:

- ✓ Pharmaceutical companies are considered to be one of the most lucrative businesses in the 21st Century.

✓ The number of hospitals has grown these past decades exponentially. Before it was believed to be due to baby boomers or those in their retirement age, however, recent studies are showing that people tend to rely more on doctors nowadays for every aspect of their physical health.

✓ Insurance rates and coverage have grown too high partly due to inflated medical and prescriptions cost.

Obviously, not all drugs are dangerous. Many have their purpose in life are beneficial to our society. However, some drugs are harmful in some ways as they are harsh and carry deadly side effects in many ways.

Nonetheless, millions of people are still choosing to forego using medications with dangerous side effects and instead resort to the holistic and natural treatment of high blood pressure. With holistic treatment, we refer to the kind of healing that view the wholeness of a person. That is, instead of focusing on the treatment of a disease, the holistic approach looks at an individual's overall physical, emotional, mental, and spiritual well being before recommending treatment.

This holistic approach to natural treatment might involve a nutritional diet, regular exercise, meditation, and much more. Attacking high blood pressure on many different angles can completely cure the person without the use of drug medication!

HOW CAN ONE BENEFIT FROM THE NATURAL TREATMENT?

Beside from the avoidance of the life-threatening side effects of drugs, there are various reasons why you need to consider treating high blood pressure naturally.

Here are some things you should consider doing:

- *WEIGHT LOSS*

    People who undergo natural treatments learn not only how they are cured of their high blood pressure, but also managed to shed extra pounds. When you know the right kind of food to eat, you will minimize your cravings and therefore can lose 1-2 pounds in a week.

- *IMPROVED STAMINA AND ENERGY*

    Because of proper nutrition, you will experience improved stamina and energy and therefore can do things that you can enjoy. When one has a healthy body, life can be better compared to those who don't have a healthy and fit body.

- *REVIVING YOUTHFULNESS*

  When you have high blood pressure, you are missing out on significant vitamins and minerals that are needed by the body. Vitamins and minerals like calcium, magnesium, and zinc play a vital role in normalizing your blood pressure. When you have adequate of these substances, then you will feel much younger and alive.

- *CONTROLLING HYPERTENSION*

  There are over a thousand listed benefits for exercising and controlling your blood pressure is one of them. Learn a simple exercise, which you can do every day for 20-30 minutes, and you will eventually experience that your blood pressure is going back to normal.

- *NO SIDE EFFECTS!!!*

  Unlike medicine drugs, the only side effect you can get from taking natural remedy is feeling bad about not trying it sooner.

NATURAL WAYS TO CONTROL HIGH BLOOD PRESSURE WITHOUT MEDICATION

Changing lifestyle is said to show a normalized blood pressure in around 86 percent of those who have this disease. Therefore, if you want to reverse your hypertension, you need to normalize your weight. Once you begin to have healthier eating habits, then you can start adapting to the following strategies to beat your hypertension.

- *STEP #1 – WALK, WALK, WALK!*

  Start to walk as much as you can. Work up to walk slowly for longer and longer distances. Try power walking – brisk walking for about 30 minutes a day. This activity can increase your oxygen supply in the body to keep your heart function smoothly and efficiently. As you get used to power walking, try to increase your speed and distance while you increase strength and stamina.

- *STEP #2 – INHALE, EXHALE!*

  Take time to breathe deeply. Sit in a chair with your back straight. Breathe as deeply as you can for five or ten minutes. Stress hormones elevate a kidney enzyme called renin, which raises blood pressure. By slowly deep breathing and expanding your belly, you exhale all the tension out of your body. Adding qigong, tai chi, meditation or yoga to that deep breath is another excellent stress buster.

- *STEP #3 – TAKE MORE POTASSIUM, REDUCE SODIUM IN YOUR DIET*

  Watch out for the amount of animal protein in your diet because overeating some of it causes a rise in your body acid levels and diminishes your potassium level. Therefore, it is better to add more naturally potassium-rich foods to your meals such as fresh fruits and vegetables, whole grain, dairy and poultry products, meat, and fish.

High potassium-rich foods include broccoli, halibut, tuna, spinach, parsley, oranges, bananas, avocados, strawberries, crimini mushrooms, Brussels sprouts, kidney beans, tuna, eggplant, apricots, dried prunes, raisins, cantaloupe, honeydew melon, potatoes, peas, squash, chard, sweet potatoes, bell peppers, cucumbers, tomatoes, and cabbage.

Buy as little processed food and limit your sodium intake by buying food that contains a higher level of sodium. You can avoid this by reading food labels, as you will become more aware of the amount of salt in every pack of food that you buy in the grocery store or supermarket. People with high blood pressure are sometimes salt-sensitive. Because there is no available test to show if you are sensitive to salt or not, it is, therefore, essential to be aware of how much salt you are taking so to be able to reduce as much as possible.

- *STEP #4 – ADD COCOA TO YOUR DIET*

A half an ounce of dark chocolate added to your diet contains at least 70 percent cocoa. Dark chocolate contains a substance called "flavanols", which make blood vessel more elastic. The elasticity of blood vessels helps to lower down high blood pressure.

Cocoa flavanols are bioactive derived from cacao beans. Studies on cacao beans disclosed that flavanols could improve cardiovascular functions while lowering the burden on the heart that comes along with aging and heart's stiffening. The study further reveals that the intake of cocoa flavanols reduces the risk of developing cardiovascular diseases.

- *STEP #5 – ALCOHOLIC BEVERAGE HELPS, TOO!*

Having about ¼ -1/2 drink of alcoholic beverage helps to lower your blood pressure. Studies revealed that a small amount of alcoholic drink in a day decreases the risk of heart disease and protects the heart. However, more than that is sure to be detrimental.

- *STEP #6 – AVOID CAFFEINE*

Studies about caffeine show that it causes high blood pressure by tightening blood vessels. This highlights the effects of stress and raises high blood pressure as well. Therefore, you can avoid a blood pressure spikes when you are stressed by using decaf coffee and other drinks.

Drinking hibiscus coffee is associated with a significant decrease in hypertension. A study has proven that drinking 3 cups of hibiscus coffee a day for six weeks brings a substantial change in the level of blood pressure of participants. The Journal of Nutrition had published that hibiscus tea can cause the blood pressure to lower down naturally and was effective in adults who are classified as either mildly hypertensive or pre-hypertensive.

- *STEP #7 – AVOID WORKING TOO MUCH!*

  Working for more than 41 hours in a week can add hypertension to the list of health risks since people who works too much tend to eat less healthy food and do not have enough time to exercise. Overload of responsibilities and tasks adds stress to your daily routine, which could later bring you more health issues. Therefore, try to rest as often as you can.

MORE ALTERNATIVE TREATMENTS TO INCLUDE IN YOUR DIET!

There are many other ways to normalize your high blood pressure, and you can include these in your diet. Here are some of them.

- *SELENIUM*

  Selenium, copper, and zinc are just some of the compound elements that can be helpful. Many studies show how people with heart diseases are often deficient of these items. You can have supplements some of these features by taking multi-vitamins in your diet. Sources of selenium are meat, walnuts, Brazil nuts, dark greens, and wheat. Zinc is usually found in beans, meat, and dairy while copper is present in seafood, legumes, nuts, and dark, leafy vegetables.

- *BETA-GLUCAN*

  This substance lowers cholesterol level and likewise reduces blood pressure resulting from high cholesterol. You can get beta-glucan from oat bran and maitake mushroom. This element further aids in moving waste materials out of the human body. A 200-milligram of oat bran (about a teaspoon) to be taken daily can lower hypertension.

- *L'ARGINE*

  By taking 2 grams of L'argine a day can reduce systolic pressure by 20 points after you have taken the supplement for two days. It is primariy due to the amino acid that helps the body to produce nitric acid, which regulates blood pressure and cholesterol.

- *FISH OIL OR FLAXSEED*

  Known as Omega 3 fatty acid, fish oil is beneficial for those who are suffering from hypertension. Fish oil protects the heart as well as lowers the blood pressure. For vegetarians, you can try flaxseed. Consuming just a tablespoon of the flaxseed daily can help you lower down your hypertension by nine points.

CHAPTER 6: HERB REMEDIES: HOW CAN THEY HELP TO NORMALIZE YOUR BLOOD PRESSURE

One of the naturally accepted treatments for high blood pressure is the use of herbal as home remedies. The recent increase in the movement away from drug medication is mainly because of the fact that people are fed up with the side effects resulting from the use of drug medication, not to say the costly prescriptions.

HERBAL REMEDIES FOR HIGH BLOOD PRESSURE

* *ARJUNA (TERMINALIA ARJUNA)*

The Arjuna plant is associated with high blood pressure treatment. Its bark is known for its remarkable remedy of the sickness by protecting the heart and stopping the bleeding as well as toughening the muscles in the organ while improving the blood circulation.

Triterpene Glycosides and *Coenzymes Q10* compound substances that help the heart and the arterial blood vessels to function properly are said to be abundant in Arjuna plant. Regular use of this herbal medicine will help eliminate the risk of hypertension and prevent further damage to the heart and the rest of vital organs that are affected by high blood pressure.

- *DANDELION (TARAXACUM OFFICINALE)*

  If you have an issue on fluid retention, dandelion can be useful as it helps increase the urine flow and helps lower blood pressure. One can benefit from the use of dandelions through the elimination of potassium loss, which pharmaceutical diuretics often have. However, make sure that when you use these dandelion leaves, they are not treated with pesticides.

- *CAYENNE (CAPSICUM ANNUM)*

  Cayenne aids in thinning of the blood, thus lowering your blood pressure. Just use the hot Mexican or Thai seeds like those used in Serrano or African Bird Peppers, which are among the hottest of the cayenne products.

  To use cayenne for remedy, just take a cup of lukewarm water mixed with one teaspoon of cayenne pepper. Drink the solution for maintenance.

- *GINGER (ZINGIBER OFFICINALE)*

Another herb that is commonly used as a cooking spice is ginger. Though we often consume this home kitchen ingredient, yet most are not aware of its health benefits, including regulating high blood pressure. Ginger is very useful in improving blood flow, treating nausea, relaxing muscles of the arteries, facilitating easy digestion, and easing morning sickness.

Garlic may come in various forms including dry roots, capsules, fresh roots, oils, liquid extracts, powders, supplements, etc. You can eat garlic raw or add it to your delectable dishes.

While ginger is proclaimed as safe and effective for hypertension, some people may experience some possible side effects which you must be cautious of – Allergic reactions, gastric disturbance, heartburn problems or mouth irritation.

• GUGGUL (COMMIPHORA WIGHTII)

Primarily, this herb grows in India but can also be found in other countries in Central Asia and Northern Africa. Studies indicate that this amazing herb can reduce bad cholesterol LDL and likewise address health issues related to psoriasis, arteriosclerotic vascular disease, and cardiac ischemia.

• GARLIC (ALLIUM SATIVUM)

For a long time, we have recognized garlic as an aromatic ingredient we used for food seasoning. However, we failed to realize that garlic lowers down our blood pressure by ten percent. Even when it's in the form of gel capsules, garlic still has the same effect.

Garlic also possesses the capability to lessen blood clotting and clears your arteries of bad cholesterols and plaques. For better performance, daily consumption of 1 or 2 cloves for 90 days is enough to prevent and minimize the effects of high blood pressure. It can either be eaten raw or included in your meals.

- *REISHI (GANODERMA LUCID)*

This is one species of mushroom associated with lowering of blood pressure. The mushroom is almost inedible but available in capsule form.

- *HAWTHORN (CRATAEGUS APP)*

  Hawthorn causes arterial walls to relax and dilate, and it can take many weeks or months to show any effect.

- *HAWTHORN (CRATAEGUS LAEVIGATA)*

  Hawthorn is beneficial in widening arterial blood vessels, preventing the growth of atherosclerosis, decreasing cholesterol levels, enhancing blood circulation, and regulating heartbeat.

  You can consume this herb by drinking it in tea form using its dried leaves and flowers. You may also include hawthorn berry supplements in your dietary plan. Whatever way you use, you can experience a 2.60 HG reduction in your blood pressure level. All these results established hawthorn as a highly trusted herbal treatment for blood pressure.

- *CELERY (APIUM GRAVEOLENS)*

Celery has been used as a remedy since the early age, and it occupies a unique herbal treatment for blood pressure. It aids in increasing the flow of urine. Indians have used it in their daily life having recognized celery as one of the best remedies for high blood pressure.

- *COCOA (THEOBROMA CACAO)*

Another fantastic herb that is associated with lowering high blood pressure efficiently is the Cocoa. It works as antioxidants like tea and red wine. According to researchers, a daily dose of 3.5 ounces of cocoa is effective as taking a daily dose of high blood pressure medication.

- *VALERIAN (VALERIANA OFFICINALIS)*

  Valerian relaxes the smooth muscles lining the arterial walls by preventing them from constricting.

- *BROCCOLI (BRASSICA OLERACEA VAR. ITALICA) AND DARK LEAFY GREENS*

  Broccoli and dark leafy vegetables are high in vitamins and minerals that are an essential need for people with high blood pressure. Magnesium and calcium are found in abundance in broccoli and other dark leafy vegetables.

- ### TURMERIC (LUCUMA LONGA)

  Turmeric, the spice, is often used in curries. It has anti-inflammatory and antioxidant properties that lower cholesterol level and strengthen body vessels as well as reduce blood pressure.

- ### GINGKO BILOBA

  Gingko Biloba is known Chinese herbal remedy for hypertension that improves circulation of the blood and dilates arteries. It also enhances memory and makes one mentally alert.

- ### OLIVE LEAF EXTRACT

  The extract derived from the olive leaf is used as a remedy for high blood pressure to combat irregular heartbeat or what is called "arrhythmia."

- *JAUNDICE BERRY*

  With this herbal remedy, blood flow is facilitated to run smoothly in the arteries by dilating blood vessels through the release of tension on the arteries.

- *CAYENNE*

  Cayenne is known as the best herb for high blood pressure next to garlic. To get the best results, choose the hottest of the cayenne spices. Cayenne is known to result in proper control of blood pressure.

- *RED CLOVER*

  People with high blood pressure tend to have their blood thickened resulting to the extra effort of the heart in pumping blood through the vessels. The pressure therefore against the arteries is heightened causing hypertension. Red clover is best for thinning blood hence, lowering blood pressure, and improving blood circulation. To be efficiently used, the red clover needs to be in good state – blossoms must remain purple. Brown coloured clover is dry and has lost their effectiveness.

- *ALFALFA*

Alfalfa helps in softening hardened arteries while reducing high blood pressure. It plays a vital role in hypertension treatment.

- *PARSLEY*

Parsley is best in maintaining blood circulation and the whole circulatory system of the body while it lowers high blood pressure.

- *GOOSEBERRY*

  Known as "Amla" in India, gooseberry can be consumed with honey in its juice form. Take 1-2 tablespoon daily on an empty stomach as is a primarily beneficial to people with high blood pressure.

- *ONION AND HONEY*

  A mixture of onion juice and honey can do wonders for people with high blood pressure. Drinking two teaspoons a day of this mixture can reverse the effect of high blood pressure and helps you return to a stable blood pressure.

- *FENUGREEK SEED (TRIGONELLA FOENUM-GRAECUM)*

  Seeds from this plant are known to carry various health benefits including the following:

- LOWERS BLOOD CHOLESTEROL

  Studies have proven that fenugreek helps in reducing cholesterol level, particularly that of LDL or low-density lipoprotein. The herb is known to be enriched with steroidal saponins, which is associated with the absorption of cholesterol and triglycerides.

- REDUCES RISKS OF HEART DISEASE

  Fenugreek leaves contain a high amount of potassium that counters the adverse effects of sodium in the body to help control heartbeat rate and blood pressure.

- KEEPS YOU IN SHAPE

    When you include fenugreek in your diet by
    chewing soaked seeds in the morning on an
    empty stomach, the natural fiber in the
    fenugreek can fill up and causes your stomach
    to swell, suppressing your appetite. This aids
    you in attaining your weight loss goals, as you
    also tend to lose your cravings for foods.

All the above conditions are beneficial and will help
you naturally lower your high blood pressure.

Chapter 7: Stress Management: Empowering Mind and Body

It's still debatable whether long-term blood pressure and stress are connected. However, taking measures to manage and reduce your stress dramatically benefits your overall health including your blood pressure.

The Connection Between Stress and Long-term High Blood Pressure

While experts cannot define the direct relationship between these two, it's proven that stressful events can cause temporary increase in blood pressure. What you can do to avoid long-term high blood pressure is to take preventive measures that will benefit your health in both mind and body.

Exercising is a drug-free way of helping you lower your blood pressure. It reduces your stress levels as it releases endorphins, which are essential in making you feel good about yourself and the things around you. For instance, you can exercise 3-5 times a week for about half an hour to reduce your stress level. Other physical activities such as doing household chores, gardening, dancing, swimming, or jogging can also increase your breathing and heart rates, generating benefits in rendering your blood pressure under control.

Remember that under stressful situations, your body produces a rush of hormones, which can cause your heart to beat faster for a while and narrowing your blood vessels in the process. As we mentioned earlier, there's no absolute proof that stress directly results in long-term blood pressure but behaviours such as overeating, smoking, substance abuse and observing poor sleeping habits can all contribute to high blood pressure. Overtime, these series of temporary sharp increases in blood pressure can put you in danger of having a long-term high blood pressure.

On the other hand, stress-related health conditions such as isolation, anxiety, and depression, which can be connected to heart disease may not be related to high blood pressure at all. The reason may be because of the hormones that are produced during the stressful moments.

These hormones can then damage the arteries, exposing you to the risks of heart disease. Additionally, if you are stressed or depressed, you also tend to neglect yourself. This includes the probability of not taking necessary medications that can control your high blood pressure and heart condition.

ACTIVITIES THAT CAN REDUCE BLOOD PRESSURE

Stress management is a skill that can help you in a lot of ways. Mastering it can help you live a healthy lifestyle that can benefit your overall health—both mind and boy—including the regulation of your blood pressure. The following steps may help you get started in how to handle your stress:

MAKE YOUR SCHEDULE SIMPLE

One of the most challenging things most of us experience is how to simplify our schedule. Usually, we tend to procrastinate only to find ourselves in a rush to finish our work, projects, assignments, etc. With this hustle and bustle, it's quite reasonable that our body accepts this as stress, which isn't good for our body when accumulated over time.

Eliminate or curtail additional activities that take up a lot of your time. For example, chatting with your friends on Facebook takes a great deal of your morning schedule. Instead of doing this, you can choose a more time-worthy activity wherein you can move around your body or exercise your mind, such as trying to meditate.

BE CONSCIOUS OF YOUR BREATHING

Breathing is essential for us; after all, we breathe to live. When we breathe, each cell in our body takes in the supply of oxygen that contributes to the production of energy in our system. It also allows us to get rid of the toxins that our body must eliminate to stay healthy.

Unfortunately, most of us take breathing for granted. Busy schedule and fast-paced lifestyle contribute more to our neglect in taking deep breaths which are very important in our health.

You can do simple breathing exercises by doing deep inhalation and exhalation all throughout the day. Take a few deep breaths and let your body relax, letting go of the stressors accumulating in your body. This process allows you to intake oxygen and feeds the cells of your body the much-needed supply necessary for your survival.

Do Regular Work Out

In this modern age wherein computers and various gadgets dominate our lifestyle, we tend to be sedentary. Remember that physical activity is a natural stress reliever. With the advice of your doctor, you can plan your exercises starting from simple activities such as walking or jogging. You can also try these various activities:

- Doing household chores and gardening
- Climbing the stairs
- Walking (in the park or any relaxing place)
- Dancing
- Playing tennis, basketball, or dodgeball

MEDITATE

Meditation has been proven to benefit the health of both our mind and body. It helps us to relax and have that inner calm that is essential to achieving balance.

Back in 2008, Massachusetts General Hospital doctor Randy Zusman asked his patients with high blood pressure to undertake a three-month-long meditation-base relaxation program. These patients regularly took medication to control their high blood pressure. After three months, 40 out of 60 patients displayed a remarkable drop in their blood pressure levels.

As a result, they were able to lessen their medication intake. The scientific explanation about this is that as the body and mind enter the state of relaxation, nitric oxide can then be formed resulting in the opening of blood vessels, regulating the flow of blood pressure.

Yoga helps you to control your blood pressure. In doing regular stretches, your muscles can become flexible resulting in controlled blood pressure without the use of medications. Stretching exercises develop a series of physiological reactions that may inhibit the stiffening of arteries due to aging.

DEVELOP GOOD SLEEPING HABITS

When you are deprived of sleep, you usually gain weight due to the lowering of your *leptin* (the hormone in charge of prompting your brain that you already had enough food eaten) hormone levels and an increase of the biochemical called *ghrelin* which intensifies your appetite to eat.

This bodily reaction dramatically affects your eating behavior, making you intake high amounts of calories which your body doesn't need.

Additionally, sleep deprivation also makes your body release higher levels of insulin after you eat, boosting fat storage and exposing you to a higher risk of having type-2 diabetes.

Sleep plays a vital role in repairing and healing your blood vessels as well as your heart. Lack of it promotes high blood pressure, stroke and heart disease.

According to one study of Harvard Medical School, patients with high blood pressure may experience the hike of their blood pressure levels all throughout the next day upon staying late the night before. To help yourself fight off sleep deprivation, here are the best steps that you should observe:

- Consume caffeine only in mornings.

- Set aside your mobile devices and other gadgets after dinner.

- Observe a consistent wake-up schedule.

- Avoid using sedatives like Valium, Nyquil, Ambien or even alcohol.

- Take a 15-minute nap every afternoon instead of drinking coffee.

BE OPTIMISTIC

Having a positive mindset and attitude dramatically helps in promoting your overall health. When you're mind is relaxed, your body automatically creates balance and harmony leading to good health—and regulating your blood pressure levels is one of the benefits of having this inner calm. Quite some studies also show that being optimistic tend to give a person a quality and long life. For instance, a happy and contented person who enjoys laughing in the company of his loved ones manages to lead a long life compared to those who suffer depression or have a negative outlook on life.

According to some studies, there is an association between the positive outlook and lower blood pressure. Individuals who have a positive mindset tend to have controlled blood pressure levels; whereas, those who look towards life in a negative perspective have the highest risk of developing high blood pressure. Moreover, positive individuals have the lower percentage of exposing themselves into evolving into cardiovascular disease.

Therefore, if you want to enjoy a quality life until your old age, it's time to recreate your mindset. You can always start with little things. In other words, you can marvel at the little things nature gives us like the sunlight, warmth, the sky or even the moon during the night.

Be conscious of your inner voice and how you talk to yourself. Avoid talking about your mistakes or highlighting your worries. Before you are tempted to do that, give yourself some space and assess the situation. While you can see unfavorable aspects, you always have the choice to shed on that matter. Don't forget to laugh in every chance you have. A good one can help lessen your mental burden, even making it easier for you to handle challenging problems.

CHAPTER 8: HOW MEDITATION CAN HELP IN LOWERING HIGH BLOOD PRESSURE

In addition to the conventional methods of combating high blood pressure, Mindfulness-Based Reduction Technique (MBRS) is gaining followers and practitioners all over the world. By incorporating mindfulness meditation into your lifestyle along with physical fitness activity and weight management, your goal of reducing high blood pressure is achieved and thereby reverse its effect on your body.

According to a research study, to curb blood pressure and ward off hypertension, it is critical to keep your mind away from stress and anxiety.

Researchers from Case Western University School of Medicine conducted a study on hundred of patients with hypertension aging 30-60 years old. The program consisted of 8 sessions covering 2 ½ hours each. Participants were then asked to meditate using the body scan exercise for 45 minutes in six days per week. The study resulted in a significant outcome with the result indicating a 1.9-mm Hg decrease in diastolic blood pressure (DBP) and 4.8-mm Hg decrease in systolic blood pressure (SBP). The findings were published in the Psychosomatic Medicine Journal.

In a recent study on blood pressure, distress and coping, it was revealed that through a selected mind-body intervention, a decrease in blood pressure was detected relative to increased coping and decreased psychological distress in young adults conducive to high blood pressure.

Based on these studies, it was proven that meditation could be useful in lowering the level of blood pressure while combating the ill effects of stress and anxiety in the human body.

As you resolve to shift to a healthier lifestyle choice, you must incorporate meditation into your everyday routine. Making a habit of practicing daily or doing meditation exercises even for just 20 minutes is sure to make a big difference on how your body moves, how your mind thinks, and how your body feels.

When your mind and emotions are calm and controllable, you're in a better position to face all the challenges in your life and the goals that you have set for yourself – which in this case happens to be regulating your blood pressure to a reasonable level.

Those negative feelings including worry, anxiety, and fear plus the regular occurrence of stress as you are regularly exposed to various stressors can be significantly relieved by a daily practice of meditation. As your mind is cleared of muddled thoughts, keeping you stuck in unhealthy behaviors, you will be surprised to see how you would see life in a different viewpoint. All the changes in your life always begin in your mind.

Your mind always has the power over your body – from the tip of your hair down to the tip of your toes.

Being able to control your mind and tame it so you can lead it to where you want is an efficient way of calming your overall sense so as not to send your heart beating or pumping as it usually does. When you can do this, then you are getting rid of the stressors that tend to send your blood pressure up.

Rather than doing the same routine using the same mindset and results that are disappointing, meditation allows you to set the stages for some significant shift in your life, and this includes, primarily your health.

MANAGING YOUR HEALTH, SAVING YOUR LIFE!

Just as human illness is relatively stress-related, meditation works well to relieve you from stress. It likewise helps in treating illnesses. Not only mediation resolve the issue on high blood pressure or hypertension risks, but it is also associated with the relief of the following diseases:

- Skin disorders

- Mild depression

- Pre-menstrual syndrome and dysmenorrhea

- Sleeping apnea and fatigue

- Recurring pain including headaches

- Respiratory issues like asthma and emphysema

- Rheumatoid Arthritis (RA) symptoms

- Gastrointestinal distress

- Irritable bowel syndrome

Health and medical condition like the ones we have here will undoubtedly deprive you of the vitality and live a life of fun and enjoyment. When you let stress weight you down as you are burdened with anxiety and negative thoughts and emotions, it stresses that is in control and not you!

Could there be more satisfying than having a cure for a stress-related illness that is natural? This is what meditation is offering you – A life of happiness – free from the claw of this deadly sickness.

A WAY TO DO YOUR MEDITATION EXERCISE

To start, find a comfortable place to do your exercise. Though old-timers can do it anywhere and would find it easy to achieve their meditation goal anywhere and anytime, beginners can get easily distracted; hence, you need a more quiet and serene place to meditate. You can either sit on a chair or the floor as long as you feel comfortable and relaxed. If you need something to soothe your senses, prepare some music.

Start by closing your eyes or just focus your attention on something like maybe the floor near where you are sitting. Then start breathing in and out gently, trying to feel the air as it passes through your nostrils and runs through every part of your body before you slowly take it out through your mouth, Feel every moment – either you focus on your breathing, or you focus on the object of your attention.

If you are closing your eyes, imagine of something – an image, an object, a mantra or anything you want to connect with. If you find your mind wandering out of focus, slowly get it back to being focused without judging yourself. The goal here is to be able to control your thinking to focus on something and not get affected emotionally but just silently look at it at the present moment.

Focusing on your breathing gives you a new awareness of your life, and while you are doing this activity, you may be able to grasp a new meaning to your existence. This could be a simple and quite exercise that could last for a few minutes, but out of it, something new – an insight maybe will be revealed to you in a spur of a moment.

Short as it is, you could not imagine the benefits this meditation exercise can bring you – physically, mentally, emotionally, and spiritually. It is for this reason that more and more people resort back to transcendental or mindfulness meditation as a way of treating stress to reverse the effects of high blood pressure or minimize the risks of more severe health problems.

Ideally, set aside 15-30 minutes a day for meditation so calm down your senses and prepare them for facing the daily struggles and challenges in life. This way, your body won't feel threatened and set itself to a fight or flight mode which causes it to produce some hormonal change in your body, sending your heart to build more pressure and forcing the arterial wall to break.

There are some online resources and tools like the Insight CD System, which you can set up by yourself and so a quick meditation session for 20 minutes or more depending on your preference.

While listening to the CD, you can teach your brain to work n synchronization –that is, training your left and right side of the brain to work in consonance to create a comprehensive distribution of electrical activity and energy patterns throughout your mind instead of having it confined to limited areas. This tool is designed in agreement with the result of a study which indicates that this full brain synchronization is active at times of intense creativity, clarity, and inspiration.

To sum this up, whether you are doing meditation without the use of the Insight audio CD or any tool like this, make sure that that you incorporate the meditation exercise in your daily activities. Make this a habit, not only to regulate your high blood pressure but a part of a healthy lifestyle. It's a simple step, but its lasting result can have a profound and lasting effect on your overall physical health and mental wellbeing.

CONCLUSION

A significant number of hypertension sufferers are now getting tired of experiencing the debilitating effects of drug prescriptions and medication that most opted to resort back to the natural remedies. Now that many are asking if the natural way of treating high blood pressure works, proven studies answer this question with a big "YES!"

However, natural treatment is a holistic approach that needs to be consolidated into your lifestyle to be able to benefit from it entirely. It does not answer to only one area of your life but needs to make a thorough overhauling of your wellbeing.

Now that you have become aware of the extent that natural remedies can do to your goal of bringing down to the reasonable level your high blood pressure, you can use this knowledge to regulate your blood pressure and manage your hypertension to prevent the onset of other complications or more severe illnesses.

High blood pressure can be a silent killer only if you neglect to give enough attention to your lifestyle. It's not high blood that kills, but it's your failure to create a healthy lifestyle that can give you a better, safer, and longer life!

The next step is for you to **join our email newsletter** to receive updates on any upcoming new book releases or promotions. You can sign-up for free and as a bonus, you will also receive our "*7 Fitness Mistakes You Don't Know You're Making*" book! This bonus book breaks down many of the most common fitness mistakes and will demystify many of the complexities and science of getting into shape. Having all this fitness knowledge and science organized into an actionable step-by-step book will help you get started in the right direction in your fitness journey! To join our free email newsletter and grab your free book, please visit the link and signup: **www.hmwpublishing.com/gift**

Finally, if you enjoyed this book, then I would like to ask you for a favor, would you be kind enough to leave a review for this book? It would be greatly appreciated!

Thank you and good luck in your journey!

Dash Diet

The Ultimate Beginner's Guide

To Dash Diet to Naturally

Lower Blood Pressure &

Proven Weight Loss Recipes

By *Louise Jiannes*

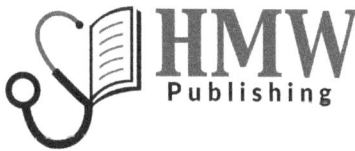

HMW Publishing

For more great books visit:

HMWPublishing.com

Table of Contents

INTRODUCTION   6

CHAPTER 1: THE MOST EFFECTIVE DIET

THAT YOU SHOULD KNOW   9

What is the DASH Diet?   10

Why was the DASH Diet created?   12

How does DASH Diet work?   14

Who should be on the DASH diet?   16

CHAPTER 2: HOW TO BE ON A

SUCCESSFUL DASH DIET   18

Tip 1: Consult your doctor regularly. (Know what you

    can get from it)   19

Tip 2: Make food that you like eating   21

Tip 3: Don't overthink about it (Routine)   23

Tip 4: Follow the recipes   26

Tip 5: Make the change gradually   28

Tip 6: Reward yourself for success and don't be too

    hard when you slip-up   30

Tip 7: Move and exercise   32

Tip 8: Look for people to join you   34

Sample Recipes   **37**

- Whole-grain Pizza Margherita   39

- Beef Stroganoff   41

- Potato Skin   44

4. Seasonal Fruit Palette   48

5. Rainbow Ice Pops   50

6. Buffalo Chicken Salad Wrap   52

7. White Chicken Chili   54

8. Curried Cream of Tomato Soup with Apples   57

9. Shrimp Ceviche   60

Recommended food servings   62

Vegetables: 4 to 5 servings a day   63

Fruits: 4 to 5 servings a day   64

Dairy: 2 to 3 servings a day   66

Change to a Healthier Lifestyle 68

CHAPTER 3: THE REWARDS THAT YOU

WILL REAP 73

Prevention of Diabetes 73

On Weight Loss 77

Hypertension 79

Osteoporosis 81

Kidney Health 82

Cancer Prevention 83

CONCLUSION 84

Final Words 89

About the Co-Author 91

INTRODUCTION

In today's modern, all of us are concerned about our health more than ever before. This is due to the increase in diseases, viruses and other things that can affect how we live and how well we can continue to live the way that we want or need to. As a result of this, many new great diets have come to be. One of the most popular, if not the most popular is the DASH Diet. The DASH Diet is aimed for the prevention and cure of common diseases such as hypertension and diabetes by especially lowering sodium intake, sugars, and fats. Although it is designed for this, it has proved to be very effective for weight loss, help lower risk of osteoporosis, kidney problems, and even cancer.

This book introduces you to this reputable diet. Not only will this book make you familiar with the new most effective diet tips, but it also contains recipe samples which will be very handy for you as you begin this healthy journey of adapting the new DASH

Diet. There are also suggestions for a healthier lifestyle changes. Get closer to your dream of becoming healthier, do not miss on the possibility of realizing your potential of being a healthy and fit individual. See the best version of yourself by following the DASH Diet and taking to heart the information contained in this book.

Also, before you get started, I recommend you joining our email newsletter to receive updates on any upcoming new book releases or promotions. You can sign-up for free, and as a bonus, you will receive a free gift. Our "*Health & Fitness Mistakes You Don't Know You're Making*" book! This book has been written to demystify, expose the top do's and don'ts and to finally equip you with the information you need to get in the best shape of your life. Due to the overwhelming amount of mis-information and lies told by magazines and self-proclaimed "gurus", it's becoming harder and harder to get reliable information to get in shape. As opposed to having to go through dozens of biased, unreliable and un-trustworthy sources to get your health & fitness information. Everything you need to help you has been broken down in this book for you to easily follow and to immediately get results to achieve your desired fitness goals in the shortest amount of time.

Once again, to join our free email newsletter and to receive a free copy of this valuable book, please visit the link and signup now: www.hmwpublishing.com/gift

CHAPTER 1: THE MOST EFFECTIVE DIET THAT YOU SHOULD KNOW

Nowadays, tips about losing weight are everywhere. Especially on social media, there are so many short videos and photos that advise on the specifics of dieting. However, these health suggestions are unreliable. Despite their invalidity, a lot of people still take them as truth. It is a waste of time, if not dangerous, for individuals who quickly adapt to what the internet tells them. You will be spared from this nonsense however because you will be learning about the real deal in dieting. It is the single most effective diet that you should straight go to instead of doing trial and errors with other trending methods. We only have one body and one life. We cannot afford to experiment with our health.

What is the DASH Diet?

DASH diet is not just another baseless social trend. It is well researched and studied. In fact, doctors and other organizations such as The National Heart, Lung, and Blood Institute, the America Heart Association, the Dietary Guidelines for Americans, and the US guidelines for treatment of high blood pressure endorse it. DASH diet is a dietary approach that helps prevent hypertension, lessen cholesterol amount in one's body, improve insulin production, and even lowers blood pressure. DASH diet goes beyond the laymen's advice of decrease sodium content in one's diet. It goes as far as designing its eating program of low fat or nonfat dairy, more fruits, and more vegetables to lower blood pressure. It stresses the importance of eating less refined grains and eat more of whole grains. DASH diet is rich in fiber, potassium, magnesium, and calcium.

Originally, DASH diet is designed to lower blood pressure and not a weight loss eating program. Mainly, it contains whole grains, fish, poultry, nuts, beans, lean meats, and moderate fat. DASH diet is comparable to the Mediterranean diet because it has particular guidelines. Due to the low sodium content of this diet on par with loads of vitamins and minerals, it does not only lower blood pressure, but it helps reduce cholesterol as well. The DASH Diet is simple and emphasizes on.

• Eating more fruits, veggies, and low-fat dairy foods

• Lessen the intake of foods that are high in cholesterol, trans-fats and saturated fat.

• Eat a moderate amount of whole grains, poultry, fish, and nuts.

• Limit intake of sweets, sodium, sugary drinks and red meats.

Why was the DASH Diet created?

The DASH Diet was not originally made to reduce unwanted fats in your body. It was however created to help people such as ourselves to live healthier and support us have lower chances of getting diseases. To be specific, this kind of diet can help you prevent hypertension, reduce cholesterol, improve insulin sensitivity and it has been proven to lower blood pressure to a healthy level. Also, this diet became more popular due to the added benefit of actually losing weight while still eating a decent amount of food that is chosen more carefully. As mentioned earlier, you can even eat meat to maintain a balanced protein intake. This will help you keep or gain muscle while losing weight in the process. Another thing that this diet does is it enables you to avoid eating "empty carbs."

Empty carbs are carbohydrates that lack the right amount of fiber. Refined grain carbohydrates are considered to be unhealthy in that sense. Some of these are food made from white flour such as cakes, cookies, white bread, etc. Bad carbohydrates can also come from taking in soft drinks, alcohol and even white rice. It is better to eat whole grains, nuts, vegetables, fruits and other things that are sources of good carbohydrates. It is important to mention that this diet is not a "low-carb" diet, it just makes you eat the good kinds of carbohydrates because carbohydrates are the body's primary source of energy thus making it very important for proper functioning.

How does DASH Diet work?

In the years 2011 up to 2015, DASH Diet has been ranked by the US News and World Report as the number one diet. Many people followed this diet. Natural remedies and a healthy diet are believed to be the best prevention and cure for illnesses including hypertension and diabetes. The effect of DASH Diet to one's body is similar to what pricey prescriptions do. Medicines can lower blood pressure and lessen the likelihood of someone experiencing a heart attack, stroke, or heart failure. The DASH diet has a similar effect on your health.

Even though you do not have hypertension and other illnesses, it is still advisable to follow the DASH Diet to prevent yourself from acquiring diseases. If you suspect yourself to be suffering from hypertension, consult your doctor immediately and inquire if you can just follow the DASH Diet instead of taking medications. On the other hand, if you are someone with hypertension and is already on prescriptions, talk to your doctor whether you can switch to

DASH Diet and gradually take yourself off the medication.

Who should be on the DASH diet?

The DASH Diet also adapts to the person's personal preferences in the sense that it also has a diet plan for people who are vegetarians, omnivores or people who want an all natural [meaning additive free] diet. There is even an option to create your DASH Diet weight loss plan with the help of their books "The DASH Diet Action Plan" and "The DASH Diet Weight Loss Solution" Basically; anyone and everyone can use it. Young or old, broad or slim. However, you may be there is no doubt that you can, and you should follow this diet plan if you want to achieve positive results. Additionally, it is recommended for people who are suffering from hypertension or pre-hypertension.

These are only some of the reasons why the DASH Diet is very popular and why it has been ranked as the number 1 diet by the US News and World report for 5 years, namely 2011, 2012, 2013, 2014 and 2015. It is also recommended by multiple groups and associations such as "The National Heart, Lung and Blood Institute," "The American Heart Association," "The Dietary Guidelines for Americans," and "US Guidelines for Treating High Blood Pressure."

In 2017, the DASH Diet was also ranked yet again as the best diet for the 7th year in a row once again by the US News and World Report.

CHAPTER 2: HOW TO BE ON A SUCCESSFUL DASH DIET

Following a diet isn't that easy. Adopting a new one is even more difficult. It requires a tremendous amount of patience and discipline to pull off. It takes a lot of guts and adjustments to make a new healthy habit. Proper diets do not just last for 1 or 2 weeks more so less than that. At least a new eating regime gets noticeable positive change by 4 or 5 weeks. Starting and finishing a proper diet takes at the very least a month and can reach a few years or even more. In this chapter, you will learn tips on how it will be easier for you to follow the DASH Diet and eventually become a healthier and stronger you. Sounds good right? Here are some tips that you can do to kick-start your new DASH Diet easily.

Tip 1: Consult your doctor regularly. (Know what you can get from it)

It is not true that anyone can do all diets and that all foods are healthy. Sometimes taking on a specific diet may cause more harm than good to a person if he or she undergoes that process. So the best thing to do before you start dieting is to consult your doctor. There is nothing wrong with knowing more about your body. It is also most definitely better if you find out if the diet program will be beneficial or detrimental to your health. There are so many things to consider regarding what diet is best for a person such as your own goals, underlying condition, fat percentage, stress levels, and metabolism. Your doctor can find these things out for you and recommend you a more specific plan for your health like particular food and when to eat them. Even meditation can be recommended if you are a stressed individual and it has affected your diet. Although it may sound like a spoon-feeding step, it would make it easier for you to begin your new diet when you are equipped with all the information you need. General guidelines may not work for your specific body type, lifestyle, goals, etc., so that is why it is best to be enlightened by your physician with a personalized diet plan with Dash Diet as its foundation.

Tip 2: Make food that you like eating

Whoever said that dieting had to be a terrible experience? Most people associate taking on a new healthy diet as some excruciating experience – not being able to eat anything tasty, being hungry all the time, feeling weak, not being ready to eat with friends and family, and being a tedious person in a group who orders the dull side of the menu. Well, only those who do not know how to be creative with their diets say that. There are hundreds of thousands of things that you could do to make your diet better and exciting. Just because you are eating healthy does not mean that it has to taste bad or it has to have no taste at all. If you put flavor into your diet meals, it will make it easier for you to continue dieting without falling out of motivation.

In addition to that, the DASH Diet comes with multiple recipes already prepared for you. Also, as previously mentioned, you can still take the option of making your recipe while still following the DASH Diet. Your confidence in your meals affects how enjoyable it is. If you keep having negative thoughts that the new food you are eating is not delicious or that you would rather have something else, then you would not taste its goodness. And your hesitation will reflect on your face, and people would start to believe that your new diet is putting you on punishment. Cheer up, be positive, and be strong. The taste may be entirely different at first, but it would not kill you – your whining would stress and kill your aspiration. So give the new meals a chance and cherish its taste before complaining or judging entirely that it tastes awful. You need to work on your positivity and mental prowess for everything in your life to go one direction towards your goal, which in this case is a healthier you.

Tip 3: Don't overthink about it (Routine)

Sometimes what makes dieting hard is the constant thought that you are dieting. It makes you feel as though you are "suffering" because you cannot eat or drink some of the things that you want or that you usually consume. In this case, it might be soft drinks or white rice or anything that was prescribed as a "do not eat" item. One way to deal with this is to stop yourself from thinking that you are dieting. Condition yourself to believe that the diet is a part of your daily life. Make it a routine. Soon after that, you will realize that you have been following the diet for so long, but you haven't thought about it anymore. It is also a right way of getting rid of bad eating habits.

According to research, it takes about 30 days to adopt a new practice. It may be difficult at first. However, most likely by the second week of repetitively doing a new diet, it would be more relaxed and more comfortable. The new routine would integrate into your own daily life. As you consistently perform such task every day, your brain and body become wired into that activity. The new diet becomes a part of your lifestyle. If you treat DASH Diet as something healthy and be calm about it instead of continually pressing yourself for changes and sharply observing discomforts, then this new program would always feel foreign to your body. And what happens if you keep conditioning your mind that something is alien? It would reject it. Your diet will fail, and your body goals would not be achieved if you keep thinking negatively about your new diet.

Tip 4: Follow the recipes

Are you afraid you would not be able to stick to your new diet? Often, fear comes from the unknown. If you do not have enough knowledge about DASH Diet, then it is not uncommon to doubt whether you can see yourself through it or not. However, as mentioned earlier, the DASH Diet comes with recipes that you can quickly follow for your dieting needs. If you do not know or enjoy cooking your recipes, then this will be the best thing to do. This tip is similar to the second tip in a way because it tells you to choose what you eat so that you will not easily give up on the diet just because you do not like the taste or you are getting tired of eating the same thing again and again. Besides, the recipes that the DASH Diet gives are delicious and nutritious. Naturally, with the new job you are trying with a.k.a Dash Diet, your brain exerts more effort to keep up with the change. If you had to do your research and extensively plan your new meals to cook, then you would get very exhausted. If the supposedly new healthy habit makes you stressed, then it would most likely be unsuccessful or have very delayed results. To enable you to maintain high energy in resuming your daily life along the new diet, you can just get yourself coached by the supplied DASH Diet recipes. If you have these to consult every day or weekly, then you would not need to tire yourself up in coming up with new dishes in line with the diet. You merely have to follow them, eat them, and smoothly go your way towards your health goals.

Tip 5: Make the change gradually

Have you ever heard the phrase "slowly but surely?" It is better to make gradual changes that make a drastic one. Your chances of achieving your health or body goals successfully are higher if you do things in relevance to your own pace and capability. For example, if you are planning to get on the new diet such as the DASH Diet, do not abruptly change your whole eating program right then and there unless you have this history of being very flexible and adaptable to change. Before your planned overall diet change, slowly add the essentials to this diet to your current diet. You may eat a few servings of fruits and veggies every day or assimilate other parts of the DASH Diet to your daily meals until you eat more of the DASH diet food and smaller of your current diet. Make the transition smooth and not shocking to your body and taste buds. Just add more and more of the DASH Diet meals every day until you get used to it or you feel strong enough to shift to the new diet entirely. Add more of these nutritious foods gradually to make it a regular habit. Just like what people say, some things go as fast as they came. So if you change your diet too quickly, you may change back to your old diet just as swiftly also. The key to successful dieting is consistency. You may be more able to stick to the program if you gradually adapt it.

Tip 6: Reward yourself for success and don't be too hard when you slip-up

The human brain works in a reward and punishment system. Usually, an individual will go for things that made him feel positive responses such as happiness, fulfillment, or pleasure. A person tends to avoid those that make him think negativity such as sadness, discomfort, anger, and pain. You can train yourself to regard successful dieting as a rewarding experience. For example, if you have consistently stuck to your new DASH Diet for the whole week, then maybe you can treat yourself to the movies, the spa, or go shopping by the weekend. Or you could consider having a little bit of a cheat day. If you do this, you could lessen the possible stress accompanied by this change of food intake. It will condition your mind that is committed to your diet and not letting go of it despite the initial discomforts is a very significant thing. On the other hand, if ever you fall short on the consistency on your new diet, then do not be too hard on yourself. Look at the situation objectively – where could have you possibly went wrong? Examine your circumstance, know your triggers, and plan on how to overcome another setback. Learn from this mistake, and come on stronger on achieving your goals.

Tip 7: Move and exercise

DASH Diet does work. However, if you want to get results sooner or see changes in your health and body faster, then it is advisable also to get your body moving. Like all diets present in the market, moving and exercising will significantly help you in achieving your goal. Having physical activities help in boosting your metabolism and lowering your blood pressure. Especially if you are the type of person who could overthink things or you are sensitive to the discomforts brought along by the changes in your diet, then it is best for you also regularly to exercise. Doing so can help declutter your mind and make you more resilient to changes and discomforts. With the endorphins released during exercise, you become stronger mentally and physically to take on any challenge. If the new diet can make you a bit down because you cannot eat sweets or fats as much as you used to, then exercising can help raise up your happy hormones and keep you off from feeling down.

Also, if you have been going to the gym, lifting some weights, going for a power run, or if you take walks in such peaceful sceneries or among people who are also trying to stay healthy – then you would feel more motivated. If you keep to your routine of school or work, then go back to your home to face your new diet and then think about what you are missing because of it, you would just feel miserable. Whereas, if you add exercise to your daily life, then you would have lesser time to self-pity or overthink things. Try to take a walk every morning. Make sure that you set aside a schedule as to when you will have your daily exercise. It does not need to be rigorous or extremely hard. The important thing is that you have physical activity. Why not try to use the stairs instead of the elevator when going to the office?

Tip 8: Look for people to join you

Both in doing a new diet plan or by starting to follow an exercise program, getting yourself a buddy proved to be effective. Unless you are uncomfortable with having a companion, this tip will be very useful in helping you continue dieting and getting healthier. How is dieting with other people help you ask? Well having other people join you, in general, is helpful because it gives you people who can support you in your efforts. You will have constant reassurance that what you are doing is worth it and that if you are having a hard time, you will have someone to help you get through it.

If you have a buddy with you, then it would not be straightforward to quit because your motivation and commitment are doubled by the two or more of you. If you have someone to do something together, then it would be easier to stick to it. For example, if you do the DASH Diet along with a friend then you can go shopping for your food or prepare your meals together. By being not alone in this, it would seem less of work and more of something fun and exciting. Usually, people would look forward to activities done together by a friend or groups of friends. And so by doing the new diet with someone would make you look forward to getting yourselves healthy. Moreover, by introducing the DASH Diet to other people, you also become a good influence and help them grow healthier people in the process. Other than assisting yourself you have also helped other people in the process.

Sample Recipes

DASH Diet is recognized by the US Department of Agriculture to be among the healthiest eating plans available to people nowadays. DASH Diet has its effectiveness acknowledged along with veganism, vegetarianism, and the Mediterranean diet. DASH Diet has been referred to by some people as the Americanized counterpart of the Mediterranean diet. Similarly, they emphasize the proper consumption of unprocessed food, whole grains, and lean meats. What sets DASH Diet apart from other preexisting diet plans is that instead of being restrictive, it is more of inclusive. Instead of a strongly inhibiting amount of calorie intake, DASH Diet promotes it. The researchers and creators of DASH Diet formulated the eating plan with foods that the people are already eating or are commonly available for them so that it would be easier for them to manage and adopt instead of eating new food or those that are hard to find in local sources.

This is where you start! You can conveniently begin your DASH Diet and be sure that you can commit to it by taking in some of these sample recipes. All the tips mentioned earlier would come in handy along these recipes. The DASH Diet presents many different recipes ranging from appetizers to beverages to main course dishes to bread dishes to desserts. Pick out the ones that are closest to the food you have in your current diet. Surely you will be able to find something that you will enjoy eating.

• Whole-grain Pizza Margherita

Ingredients

For the dough:

- 1 tsp of active dry yeast

- 3/4 cup of warm water

- ¾ cup of whole-wheat flour

- 2 tbsps of barley flour

- 2 teaspoons of gluten

- 1 tbsp of oats

- 1 tbsp of olive oil

For the topping

- 2 ½ cups of spinach, chopped

- 2 ½ cups of tomatoes, sliced

- 1 tbsp of oregano (minced)

- 1 tbsp of garlic (minced)

- 1 tsp of black pepper

- 2 ounces of mozzarella, fresh

Directions

1. To make the dough, dissolve yeast in warm water, let sit 5 minutes. Mix dry ingredients. Add oil and water-yeast mixture. Knead for 10-15 minutes for best texture. An electric mixer is helpful, but not necessary.

2. Let dough rise in the refrigerator for a minimum of 1 hour.

3. Preheat oven to 450 F. out dough ball on floured surface to 1/4-inch thickness. Place dough on baking sheet or pizza peel. Top with spinach, tomatoes, basil, oregano, garlic, black pepper, and mozzarella. Bake for 10-12 minutes, or until cheese melts and crust becomes crispy. Serve hot and enjoy.

• **Beef Stroganoff**

Ingredients

- 1/2 cup chopped onion

- 1/2 pound boneless beef round steak, cut 3/4-inch thick, all fat removed

- 4 cups uncooked yolk-less egg noodles

- 1/2 can fat-free cream of mushroom soup (undiluted)

- 1/2 cup of water

- 1 tablespoon all-purpose (plain) flour

- 1/2 teaspoon paprika

- 1/2 cup fat-free sour cream

Dircctions

1. In a nonstick frying pan, sauté the onions over medium heat until they're translucent, about 5 minutes. Add the beef and continue to cook for another 5 minutes or until the beef is

tender and browned throughout. Drain well and set aside.

2.   Fill a large pot 3/4 full with water and bring to a boil. Add the noodles and cook until al dente (tender), 10 to 12 minutes, or according to the package directions. Drain the pasta thoroughly.

3. In a saucepan, whisk together the soup, water, and flour over medium heat. Stir until the sauce thickens, about 5 minutes.

4.   Add the soup mixture and paprika to the beef in the frying pan. Over medium heat, stir the mixture until warmed through. Remove from heat and add the sour cream. Stir until combined.

5.   To serve, divide the pasta among the plates. Top with the beef mixture and serve immediately.

• **Potato Skin**

Ingredients

- 2 medium russet potatoes

- Butter-flavored cooking spray

- 1 tablespoon minced fresh rosemary

- 1/8 teaspoon freshly ground black pepper

Directions

1. Preheat the oven to 375 F.

2. Wash the potatoes and pierce with a fork. Place in the oven and bake until the skins are crisp about 1 hour.

3. Carefully — potatoes will be very hot — cut the potatoes in half and scoop out the pulp, leaving about 1/8 inch of the potato flesh attached to the skin. Save the pulp for another use.

4. Spray the inside of each potato skin with butter-flavored cooking spray. Press in the rosemary and pepper.

5. Return the skins to the oven for 5 to 10 minutes. Serve immediately.

4. Raspberry Chocolate Scones

Ingredients

- 1 cup whole-wheat pastry flour

- 1 cup all-purpose flour

- 1 tablespoon baking powder

- 1/4 teaspoon baking soda

- 1/3 cup trans-fat-free buttery spread

- 1/2 cup fresh or frozen raspberries

- 1/4 cup miniature chocolate chips

- 1 cup plus 2 tablespoons plain fat-free yogurt

- 2 tablespoons honey

- 1/2 teaspoon sugar

- 1/4 teaspoon cinnamon

Directions

1. Mix flours, baking powder and baking soda in a large mixing bowl.

2. Cut in buttery spread until crumbly.

3. Add berries and chocolate chips. Mix gently.

4. Mix yogurt and honey in a small bowl.

5. Add yogurt mixture to flour mixture, mixing until just blended.

6. Place ball of dough on the countertop. Knead one or two times.

7. Roll into a 1/2-inch-thick circle.

8. Cut into 12 wedges.

9. Place on lightly greased baking sheet.

10. Mix sugar and cinnamon in a small bowl.

11. Sprinkle over top of scones.

12. Bake at 400 F for 10 to 12 minutes.

4.   Seasonal Fruit Palette

Ingredients

- 1/4 teaspoon ground cinnamon

- 1/4 teaspoon sugar

- 2 cups frozen strawberries, unsweetened (thawed)

- 1/2 cup powdered sugar

- 1 star fruit, sliced

- 1 peach, pitted and sliced

- 1 pear, pitted and sliced

- 1 plum, pitted and sliced

- 1 kiwi, peeled and sliced

- Fresh mint leaves, for garnish

Directions

1.   In a small bowl, stir together the cinnamon and sugar. Set aside.

2.   In a food processor or blender, combine the strawberries and powdered sugar. Pulse until smooth.

3.   Pour onto chilled dessert plates that have a rim.

4.   Arrange the sliced fruit on top.

5.   Sprinkle with the cinnamon-sugar mixture.

6.   Garnish with fresh mint and serve immediately.

5.   Rainbow Ice Pops

Ingredients

•   1 1/2 cups diced strawberries, cantaloupe and watermelon

•   1/2 cup blueberries

•   2 cups 100 percent apple juice (or another favorite juice)

•   6 paper cups (6-8 ounces each)

•   6 craft sticks

Directions

1. Mix the fruit and divide evenly into the paper cups.

2.   Pour 1/3 cup of juice into each paper cup.

3.   Place the cups on a level surface in the freezer.

4.   Freeze until partially frozen, approximately 1 hour.

5.   Insert a craft stick into center of each pop. Freeze until firm.

6.   Buffalo Chicken Salad Wrap

Ingredients

- 3-4 ounces of chicken breasts

- 2 whole chipotle peppers

- 1/4 cup white wine vinegar

- 1/4 cup low-calorie mayonnaise

- 2 stalks celery, diced

- 2 carrots, cut into matchsticks

- 1 small yellow onion, diced (about 1/2 cup)

- 1/2 cup thinly sliced rutabaga or another root vegetable

- 4 ounces spinach, cut into strips

- 2 whole-grain tortillas (12-inch diameter)

Directions

1. You can use leftover or rotisserie chicken if you have it. If not, preheat oven to 375 F or start the grill.

2. Bake or grill chicken breasts for about 10 minutes on each side until interior temperature is 165 F.

3. Remove, cool and cube chicken.

4. In a blender, puree chipotle peppers with white wine vinegar and mayonnaise.

5. Place all ingredients except spinach and tortillas in a bowl and mix thoroughly.

6. Place 2 ounces spinach and half the mixture in each tortilla and wrap. Cut each wrap in half to serve.

7.   White Chicken Chili

Ingredients

- 1 can (10 ounces) white chunk chicken

- 3 cups cooked white beans

- 1 can (14.5 ounces) low-sodium diced tomatoes

- 4 cups low-sodium chicken broth

- 1 medium onion, chopped

- 1/2 medium green pepper, chopped

- 1 medium red pepper, chopped

- 2 garlic cloves, minced

- 2 teaspoons chili powder

- 1 teaspoon ground cumin

- 1 teaspoon dried oregano

- Cayenne pepper, to taste

- 6 tablespoons shredded reduced-fat

Monterey Jack cheese

- 3 tablespoons chopped fresh cilantro

- 6 ounces low-fat baked tortilla chips (about 65 chips)

Directions

1. In a large soup pot, add the chicken, beans, tomatoes and chicken broth. Cover and simmer over medium heat.

2. Meanwhile, spray a nonstick frying pan with cooking spray. Add the onions, peppers and garlic and sauté until the vegetables are soft, 3 to 5 minutes.

3. Add the onion and pepper mixture to the soup pot.

4. Stir in the chili powder, cumin, oregano and, as desired, cayenne pepper.

5.   Simmer for about 10 minutes, or until all the vegetables are soft.

6.   Ladle into warmed bowls.

7.   Sprinkle each serving with 1 tablespoon cheese and 1 teaspoon cilantro.

8.   Serve with baked chips on the side (about 6 to 8 chips with each serving of chili).

8.   Curried   Cream   of   Tomato Soup with Apples

Ingredients

- 2 tablespoons olive oil

- 1 1/2 cups finely chopped onion

- 1 cup finely chopped celery

- 1 teaspoon minced garlic

- 1 tablespoon curry powder, or to taste

- 3 cups no-salt-added canned tomatoes,

drained

- 1 bay leaf

- 1/2 teaspoon thyme

- Ground black pepper, to taste

- 1 cup long-grain brown rice

- 6 cups low-sodium vegetable or chicken

broth

- 1 cup fat-free milk

- 1 1/2 cups apple cubes

Directions

1. In a soup pot, heat the oil over medium heat.

2. Add the chopped onion, celery and garlic.

3. Saute until tender, about 4 minutes.

4. Add the curry powder and cook, stirring about 1 minute.

5. Add the tomatoes, bay leaf, thyme, black pepper, and rice.

6. Stir constantly while bringing to a boil.

7. Add broth.

8. Return to boil and then simmer for about 30 minutes.

9. When rice is tender, remove the bay leaf.

10.   Pour the soup into a food processor or blender and puree until smooth.

11.   Pour the soup back into the pot and add the milk and apple cubes.

12.   Cook until heated through.

13.   Ladle into individual warmed bowls and serve immediately.

9.   Shrimp Ceviche

Ingredients

•   1/2 pound raw shrimp, cut in 1/4-inch pieces

• 2 lemons, zest, and juice

• 2 limes, zest, and juice

•   2 tablespoons olive oil

•   2 teaspoons cumin

•   1/2 cup diced red onion

•   1 cup diced tomato

•   2 tablespoons minced garlic

•   1 cup black beans, cooked

•   1/4 cup diced serrano chili pepper and seeds removed

•   1 cup diced cucumber, peeled and seeded

•   1/4 cup chopped cilantro

Directions

1.   Place shrimp in a shallow pan and cover with juice from the lemon and lime, reserving the zest.

2.   Refrigerate for at least 3 hours or until shrimp is firm and white.

3.   Mix remaining ingredients in separate bowl and set aside while shrimp is cold cooking.

4.   When ready to serve, mix shrimp and citrus juice with remaining ingredients.

5.   Serve with baked tortilla chips.

Recommended food servings

If you are the type who likes to create your dishes, then feel free to use your creativity. Aside from the healthy recipes, here are the essentials of DASH Diet that you can use as guidelines in preparing your meals. Listed below are some suggestions from the DASH Diet and what portions you can follow:

Grains: 6 to 8 servings a day

• Grains include bread, cereal, rice, and pasta. Examples of one serving of grains include 1 slice whole-wheat bread, 1 ounce (oz.) dry cereal, or 1/2 cup cooked cereal, rice or pasta.

• Focus on whole grains because they have more fiber and nutrients than do refined grains. For instance, use brown rice instead of white rice, whole-wheat pasta instead of regular pasta and whole-grain bread instead of white bread. Look for products labeled "100 percent whole grain" or "100 percent whole wheat."

•   Grains are naturally low in fat, so avoid spreading on butter or adding cream and cheese sauces.

Vegetables: 4 to 5 servings a day

•   Tomatoes, carrots, broccoli, sweet potatoes, greens and other vegetables are full of fiber, vitamins, and such minerals as potassium and magnesium. Examples of one serving include 1 cup raw leafy green vegetables or 1/2 cup cut-up raw or cooked vegetables.

•   Don't think of vegetables only as side dishes — a hearty blend of vegetables served over brown rice or whole-wheat noodles can serve as the main dish for a meal.

• Fresh or frozen vegetables are both good choices. When buying frozen and canned vegetables, choose those labeled as low sodium or without added salt.

• To increase the number of servings, you fit in daily, be creative. In a stir-fry, for instance, cut the amount of meat in half and double up on the vegetables.

Fruits: 4 to 5 servings a day

• Many fruits need little preparation to become a healthy part of a meal or snack. Like vegetables, they're packed with fiber, potassium, and magnesium and are typically low in fat — exceptions include avocados and coconuts.

Examples of one serving include 1 medium fruit or 1/2 cup fresh, frozen or canned fruit or 4 ounces of juice.

•   Have a piece of fruit with meals and one as a snack, then round out your day with a dessert of fresh fruits topped with a splash of low-fat yogurt.

•   Leave on edible peels whenever possible. The peels of apples, pears and most fruits with pits add interesting texture to recipes and contain healthy nutrients and fiber.

• Remember that citrus fruits and juice, such as grapefruit, can interact with certain medications, so check with your doctor or pharmacist to see if they're OK with you.

• If you choose can fruit or juice, make sure no sugar is added.

Dairy: 2 to 3 servings a day

• Milk, yogurt, cheese and other dairy products are major sources of calcium, vitamin D, and protein. But the key is to make sure that you choose dairy products that are low fat or fat-free because otherwise, they can be a major source of fat — and most of it is saturated. Examples of one serving include 1 cup skim or 1 percent milk, 1 cup yogurt, or 1 1/2 oz. Cheese.

• Low-fat or fat-free frozen yogurt can help you boost the number of dairy products you eat while offering a sweet treat. Add fruit for a healthy twist.

• If you have trouble digesting dairy products, choose lactose-free products or consider taking an over-the-counter product that contains the enzyme lactase, which can reduce or prevent the symptoms of lactose intolerance.

• Go easy on regular and even fat-free cheeses because they are typically high in sodium.

Lean meat, poultry, and fish: 6 or fewer servings a day

• Meat can be a rich source of protein, B vitamins, iron, and zinc. But because even lean varieties contain fat and cholesterol, don't make them a mainstay of your diet — cut back typical meat portions by one-third or one-half and pile on the vegetables instead. Examples of one serving include 1 oz. Cooked skinless poultry, seafood or lean meat or 1 egg.

• Trim away skin and fat from poultry and meat and then bake, broil, grill or roast instead of frying in fat.

• Eat heart-healthy fish, such as salmon, herring, and tuna. These types of fish are high in omega-3 fatty acids, which can help lower your total cholesterol.

These suggestions are some of the servings directly quoted from the DASH Diet. What was presented here are well-balanced amounts of servings that will help you achieve your goal of either lowering blood pressure or cutting down some weight.

Change to a Healthier Lifestyle

Dieting alone would not fully make you a healthier person. Although having a good diet creates significant improvement in your health, there is still something you can do to be even better. Or if your new diet has not been making any progress then a few lifestyle changes are advisable. For example, if you have hypertension, the cause of your condition is not only from an unhealthy diet, but it is also affected by your habits. It just makes sense that you should change not only your eating program but your other practices as well to reduce or eliminate your hypertension. Here are a few gradual changes you could apply to your life:

• Water – drink a bit more of water every day. It is recommended to consume at least 2 liters of water daily. Limit or eradicate at all drinking sugar-sweetened beverages such as sodas, chocolate drinks, sugary shakes, coffee, and the like.

• Drinking – lessen your alcohol intakes especially that most drinking sessions are associated with other unhealthy habits

- Smoking – lessen your smoking habit until you can entirely quit it. Stay away from individuals smoking or from smoking areas as to not risk yourself from breathing secondhand smoke

- Sleep – get more sleep if you are not having enough, and get proper amount of sleep if you are having too much

- Dessert – you can eat have fruits as dessert instead of the usual sugar-filled ones such as ice cream, chocolates, candies, cake, and other pastries. If you want to eat some sweets, eat in smaller portions.

- Salt – instead of using salt in your cooking, use herbs and spices instead. To avoid using salt or to limit its accessibility, do not put salt shakers on your dining table.

• Snacks – most individuals opt for salty and sweet snacks. When you start inching for another bag of potato chips or a box of doughnuts, have some fresh fruits instead. Another thing you can snack on are strips of vegetables. You can keep cut carrots, mixed greens, and bell peppers for a quick snack.

• Be more active – at least spare 10 minutes a day to exercise like walking, taking the stairs, bicycling, jogging, etc. If you can, it is better to have at least 30 minutes of work out for four to five times a week.

• Exercise plan – plot yourself an exercise plan or get yourself a work out buddy or a personal trainer to be able to stick to keeping yourself fit.

• Health check – regularly consult your physician instead of only taking a trip to the clinic if you are sick or unwell. It is best to have your blood pressure, blood cholesterol, and glucose levels checked timely.

It is not easy to make an abrupt change in your lifestyle. So try to apply one or two of them week by week until you form a habit of it. In no time, you would get used to having such healthy lifestyle, and you would just naturally be such a healthy individual.

CHAPTER 3: THE REWARDS THAT YOU WILL REAP

With the DASH Diet having its foundation on health rather than vanity, there are so many benefits that you can get when following the diet. Below are some of its great rewards to help you further understand and take that first step to changing your life for the better.

Prevention of Diabetes

It is estimated that in the United States of America alone there are 29.1 million people who have diabetes. Out of that 29.1 million 8.1 million of them may be undiagnosed or unaware of their current condition. In adults 20 and older, more than one in every 10 people suffers from diabetes, and in seniors (65 and older), that figure rises to more than one in four. Diabetes is not something to be taken lightly. A person who is affected by this condition can experience getting damage to the large blood vessels of the brain, heart or legs. Damage to the small blood vessels is also possible; this can cause problems to the eyes, kidneys, feet, and nerves. Right now there is still no cure for diabetes. With this in mind, the best thing to do is to follow the saying; "prevention is better than a cure."

There are two main types of diabetes; Type 1 and Type 2. The difference between the two is basically how they are acquired, but they have the same effect. Diabetes is caused by the increase of glucose in the blood which in turn is caused by the lack of insulin or possibly the body not responding properly to the insulin which is already present. This is where the DASH Diet plays its role. According to a study conducted by Angela D. Liese, PhD, MPH, Michele Nichols, MS, Xuezheng Sun, MSPH, Ralph B. D'Agostino, Jr., PhD and Steven M. Haffner, MD wherein they associated the occurrence of type 2 diabetes in people from different races and places and with different genders whom all followed the Dash Diet. They were able to conclude from their study that the Dash Diet may indeed prove beneficial to the prevention of diabetes.

Since this diet promotes the improvement of insulin sensitivity it also helps prevent the occurrence of diabetes in the person who follows it. According to multiple studies that tackled the effects of diet accompanied by different degrees of exercise on the occurrence of diabetes, "Previous randomized trials of lifestyle interventions have demonstrated that increasing physical activity combined with a diet to encourage weight loss can decrease the incidence of type 2 diabetes in susceptible individuals... Diet interventions focused on caloric restriction, reduced fat intake, and increased fiber consumption. Overall, the exercise plus diet interventions resulted in significant weight loss and reduced the risk of diabetes by 37%." About the DASH Diet specifically, it is clear that it is under this category since the diet will also tell you to lower your fat and sodium intake and only eat good carbohydrates rich in fiber and many other things.

On Weight Loss

Losing weight is possible when there is lesser calorie count in one's body. The DASH Diet, however, do not emphasize on reducing calorie intake. It suggests nutrient-dense foods instead of calorie-rich ones to lose some inches off the waist. Fiber-rich diet proved to be effective in losing weight.

The best way to be healthy is to have a well-balanced diet which is at the same time packed with nutrients. And the DASH Diet is absolutely that. Due to its malleability, it allows for a successful and sustainable dieting. It does not leave the body deprived and hungry, unlike other diet plans. It merely reduces the number of processed fats and sweets and reimburses with fruits, vegetables, and low-fat dairy produce. Although the DASH Diet was initially created to lower blood pressure, it is also beneficial for losing weight. It is due to its eating plan that involves real foods with the right proportion of proteins, and with lots of fruits and vegetables. Because it is healthy and smooth at the same time, it is applicable throughout one's life. It is also not restrictive on adults or individuals who have health conditions, but anyone can eat it including the kids or the whole family. With DASH diet as the household's healthy meal plan, there would be lesser or no need at all for anyone to watch their diet. This is very beneficial for individuals who are gaining weight due to metabolic syndrome, type 2 diabetes, PCOS, and postmenopausal weight gain.

Hypertension

Dash in DASH Diet means Dietary Approaches to Stop Hypertension. In the U.S. alone, hypertension affects over fifty million people. Internationally, individuals who have high blood pressure reach up to 1 billion. Reportedly by the World Health Organization, hypertension causes approximately 7.1 million deaths yearly. Hypertension is a severe case since it does not only affect one's blood pressure but it affects or causes other conditions in one's body. It induces a heart attack, stroke, heart failure, and even kidney disease. By eating the DASH Diet and sparing yourself from hypertension, you are also keeping yourself away from other circulatory and excretory diseases.

To give you a glimpse of what is a healthy blood pressure and when you should start to worry, here is a bit of an explanation regarding normal blood pressure. There are two numbers recorded as blood pressure is taken – one is systolic, and another one is diastolic. The name on top is systolic, while the bottom one is diastolic. Systolic is usually higher than diastolic. It measures the pressure in the arteries as the muscles in the heart contracts or heartbeat. On the other hand, diastolic is the number that measures the pressure in the arteries in between muscle contraction in the heart or when it is resting or refilling blood. The normal range for systolic pressure is 120 or below while the normal range for diastolic pressure is 80 or lower. So numbers higher than these imply tendency of having hypertension.

Osteoporosis

Another health benefit to DASH Diet is sparing you from having osteoporosis. It is a disease where the body produces too much or too little bones or losses bones. It is quite common among elderly individuals. The new DASH Diet can help you avoid suffering from this illness. The diet is rich in calcium, protein, and potassium which are all necessary for preventing or slowing down osteoporosis. Food such as milk, lean meat, grains, leafy vegetables, and fruits help build stronger bones. See yourself as a healthy older adult with good posture if you start eating the DASH Diet as soon as possible.

Kidney Health

Kidney problems are among the most common diseases that individuals nowadays have – from urinary tract infections (UTI), kidney stones, to kidney failure. These are caused by excessive mineral deposits in the kidneys that form into stones. It makes urinating very painful. It also creates other bodily pains such as intense backaches. High mineral deposits in one's kidneys result from high sodium intake which dehydrates the body and overworks the kidneys. DASH Diet includes lowering of sodium in one's meals, which ultimately makes it very helpful in the prevention of and recovery from kidney problems.

Cancer Prevention

One the diseases that people fear the most is cancer. Cancer is somewhat unpredictable since it could happen to anyone. However, the chances of getting one can be lowered by adopting the DASH Diet. The high concentration of fiber, vitamins, and antioxidants in fruits, vegetables, and whole grains in the DASH Diet lessens or stops altogether the effect of free radicals. One of them is the byproducts of cellular respiration. This causes mutation in healthy cells which can lead to cancer.

CONCLUSION

Undoubtedly, the DASH Diet is by far the most effective and useful eating program not just for those with body conditions but for those who are aiming to cut some pounds off their body. There are so many benefits one can get when eating the DASH Diet. Despite it being a new eating program, it proves to be less difficult to adapt to, unlike other preexisting diets. DASH Diet is very beneficial to individuals of all ages, even to the whole family. Among its main purposes are to help with:

• Hypertension or high blood pressure

• Diabetes

• Weight loss

Additionally, it is great for the alleviation and prevention of osteoporosis, kidney problems, and cancer. DASH Diet is a very nutritious eating program. To sum up, its general idea on how to eat a healthy diet, take this in mind:

• Grains and grain products: 6 to 8 servings include at least three whole grain foods such as sliced bread, dry cereal, cooked cereal, pasta, rice, or barley

•	Fruits: 4 to 5 servings such as grapefruits, banana, raisins, dried fruits

•	Vegetables: 4 to 5 servings such as spinach leaves, peppers, sliced tomatoes, sprouts, zucchini, portobello mushrooms, and eggplant

•	Low- or non-fat dairy foods: 2 to 3 servings such as 1% to nonfat milk, low-fat yogurt, and cheese

•	Lean meats, fish, poultry: 6 or less such as fresh chicken breast or legs, fresh turkey breast, loin cuts of beef, sirloin, round steak, extra-lean ground beef, pork loin roast, pork tenderloin, fresh fish, and low-sodium canned tuna

•	Nuts, seeds, and legumes: 4 to 5 servings per week such as nut butter, unsalted sunflower seeds

•	Healthy Fats: 2 to 3 servings such as olive, peanut, canola oils, soybean oil, and corn oil

•	Sweets: 2 or fewer such as a 2-inch square brownie, a

small donut, a miniature candy bar, 2 small cookies, 1 small muffin, and 1 small piece of pie or cake

By sticking to this diet, you will naturally be consuming lesser salt. If you cannot follow the suggested recipe samples in this book and you want to cook the same dishes you are used to preparing; you can limit your sodium intake by simply putting less or no salt at all on the meals you cook. Also, it would help to remove the salt shakers on your dining table, so you do not keep on adding salt to your meals. Another thing to watch besides your sodium intake is your alcohol consumption. Males should cut down their liquor to at most 2 drinks per day while females should limit herself to only one. By controlling one's alcohol consumption, one's weight would be managed better, blood pressure will be normal, and dehydration would be less likely to occur.

This DASH Diet book gives you everything you need to know to successfully be a healthier you. Besides giving you actual recipes you can use while you are still new with the diet, the book also suggested lifestyle changes you can make to be healthier, and also to aid the progress that the DASH Diet will bring upon your body. Remember these healthy habits that you should gradually incorporate into your daily life.

• Drink more water every day and cut back on sweetened and alcoholic drinks

• Quit smoking or stay away from secondhand smoke

• Snack on fruits and vegetables and just eat little portions of sweets and fats

• Use herbs and spices instead of salt; do not put salt shakers on your dining table to avoid adding more salt to your meals

• Exercise at least 10 minutes a day if you are really busy like taking the stairs, walking, or riding the bicycle

• Get a workout buddy or personal trainer so that you can do at least 30 minutes of exercise 4 to 5 times a week

• Consult with your doctor regularly

Your goal of achieving a healthier you is within your reach. DASH Diet is your best choice in going towards this aspiration. Unlike other diets, DASH Diet is directed towards preventing or alleviating certain body conditions instead of focusing on just losing weight to look good. Aim towards your core health first, and then your vigor will manifest outside with a fit body. You are not left alone to struggle hard with your initial attempt on DASH Diet because even from this book alone, you are furnished recipes and guidelines that you can use for your daily new healthy lifestyle. Try it out for a week or so, and you will know how easy it is. For sure you would quickly progress to a second, third, up to a fourth week, and up to a whole healthy lifetime.

Final Words

Thank you again for purchasing this book!

I really hope this book is able to help you.

The next step is for you to **join our email newsletter** to receive updates on any upcoming new book releases or promotions. You can sign-up for free and as a bonus, you will also receive our "*7 Fitness Mistakes You Don't Know You're Making*" book! This bonus book breaks down many of the most common fitness mistakes and will demystify many of the complexities and science of getting into shape. Having all this fitness knowledge and science organized into an actionable step-by-step book will help you get started in the right direction in your fitness journey! To join our free email newsletter and grab your free book, please visit the link and signup: **www.hmwpublishing.com/gift**

Finally, if you enjoyed this book, then I would like to ask you for a favor, would you be kind enough to leave a review for this book? It would be greatly appreciated!

Thank you and good luck in your journey!

About the Co-Author

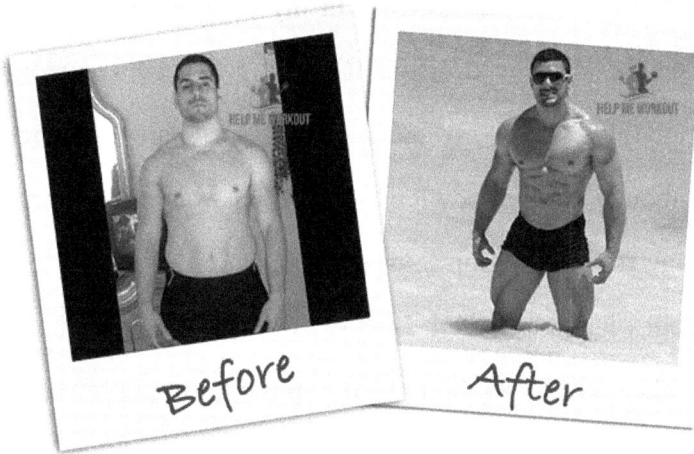

Before — After

My name is George Kaplo; I'm a certified personal trainer from Montreal, Canada. I'll start off by saying I'm not the biggest guy you will ever meet and this has never really been my goal. In fact, I started working out to overcome my biggest insecurity when I was younger, which was my self-confidence. This was due to my height measuring only 5 foot 5 inches (168cm), it pushed me down to attempt anything I ever wanted to achieve in life. You may be going through some challenges right now, or you may simply want to get fit, and I can certainly relate.

For me personally, I was always kind of interested in the health & fitness world and wanted to gain some muscle due to the numerous bullying in my teenage years about my height and my overweight body. I figured I couldn't do anything about my height, but I sure can do something about how my body looked like. This was the beginning of my transformation journey. I had no idea where to start, but I just got started. I felt worried and afraid at times that other people would make fun of me for doing the exercises the wrong way. I always wished I had a friend that was next to me who was knowledgeable enough to help me get started and "show me the ropes."

After a lot of work, studying and countless trial and errors. Some people began to notice how I was getting more fit and how I was starting to form a keen interest in the topic. This led many friends and new faces to come to me and ask me for fitness advice. At first, it seemed odd when people asked me to help them get in shape. But what kept me going is when they started to see changes in their own body and told me it's the first time that they saw real results!

From there, more people kept coming to me, and it made me realize after so much reading and studying in this field that it did help me but it also allowed me to help others. I'm now a fully certified personal trainer and have trained numerous clients to date who have achieved amazing results.

Today, my brother Alex Kaplo (also a Certified Personal Trainer) and I own & operate this publishing venture, where we bring passionate and expert authors to write about health and fitness topics. We also run an online fitness website "HelpMeWorkout.com" and I would love to connect with by inviting you to visit the website on the following page and signing up to our e-mail newsletter (you will even get a free book). Last but not least, if you are in the position I was once in and you want some guidance, don't hesitate and ask... I'll be there to help you out!

Your friend and coach,

George Kaplo

Certified Personal Trainer

Download another book for Free

I want to thank you for purchasing this book and offer you another book (just as long and valuable as this book), "Health & Fitness Mistakes You Don't Know You're Making", completely free.

Visit the link below to signup and receive it:

www.hmwpublishing.com/gift

In this book, I will break down the most common health & fitness mistakes, you are probably committing right now, and I will reveal how you can easily get in the best shape of your life!

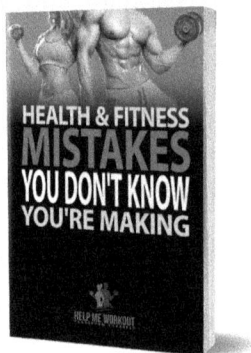

In addition to this valuable gift, you will also have an opportunity to get our new books for free, enter giveaways, and receive other valuable emails from me. Again, visit the link to sign up:

www.hmwpublishing.com/gift

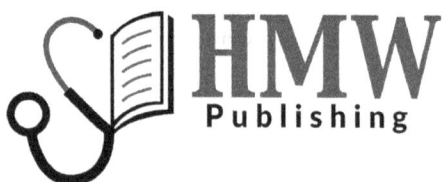

For more great books visit:

HMWPublishing.com